FROM MANAGING TO CONQUERING PULMONARY EMBOLISM

Expert Guide To Understanding the Causes, Recognizing Symptoms, Prevention and Embracing Effective Treatments for a Vibrant and Healthy Life

DR. DASHIELL DANIEL

Introduction 9
Objective Of The Book 10
Comprehending Pulmonary Embolism Is Crucial 11
The Intended Audience 12
Range And Restrictions 13

CHAPTER ONE 15

FUNDAMENTALS OF PULMONARY EMBOLISM 15
Overview Of Empathy 15
Pulmonary Embolism Types 16
The Lungs' Anatomy And Function 17
Circulation Of The Pulmonary 17
The Function Of Coagulation 18
Risk Elements For Heart Attack 19
DVT, Or Deep Vein Thrombosis 19
Additional Contributing Elements 20

CHAPTER TWO 22

ORIGINS AND PATHOPHYSIOLOGY 22
The Cause And Development Of Blood Clots 22
Common Reasons For Heart Attacks 23

CHAPTER THREE 27

CLINICAL PRESENTATION 27
Three Additional Related Symptoms 29
Diagnostic Differentiation: 29
CHAPTER FOUR DIAGNOSTIC METHODS 32
Imaging Methodologies 32
Laboratory Examinations 33

CHAPTER FIVE   36

AVAILABLE TREATMENTS   36

CHAPTER SIX   42

STRATEGIES FOR PREVENTION   42

CHAPTER SEVEN   47

INTRICACIES AND PROLONGED CONSEQUENCES   47

CHAPTER EIGHT   51

EDUCATION AND SUPPORT FOR PATIENTS   51
CONCLUSION   56

Disclaimer

This book, is intended to provide information and guidance on the subject matter and is not a substitute for professional medical advice, diagnosis, or treatment.

The author, is not a medical professional, and the content presented here is based on research, general knowledge, and expert guidance available at the time of writing.

The information in this book is provided with the understanding that the author and the publisher are not engaged in rendering medical, legal, or other professional services.

Any reliance on the information contained in this book is at the reader's own risk.

While every effort has been made to ensure the accuracy and completeness of the information presented, medical knowledge is constantly evolving, and new research may supersede the content in this book. The author and the publisher make no representations or warranties of any kind, express or implied, about the completeness, accuracy, reliability, suitability, or availability concerning the information, products, services, or related graphics contained in this book.

This book may contain references or mentions of individuals, products, websites, organizations, or other names for informational purposes only.

The author does not own or endorse any such entities mentioned in the book. Any resemblance to actual persons, living or dead, or actual events is purely coincidental.

Readers are encouraged to consult with qualified healthcare professionals for medical advice, diagnosis, and treatment tailored to their specific circumstances.

The author and the publisher disclaim any liability for any loss or risk, personal or otherwise, arising directly or indirectly from the use of the information presented in this book.

By reading this book, the reader acknowledges and agrees to the terms of this disclaimer.

In the world of medicine and healthcare, the book "Pulmonary Embolism" is extremely important since it offers a thorough and in-depth examination of a serious medical problem. This paper is significant because it provides a thorough analysis of pulmonary embolism, making it a useful tool for researchers, students, and medical professionals who want a deeper understanding of the condition.

The goal of the book is introduced in the first section, which highlights the critical necessity for a thorough investigation of pulmonary embolism. Because this disorder has the potential to be fatal, it becomes extremely important to understand its nuances; the book discusses the importance of this understanding in therapeutic practice. The insights offered are intended to help a wide range of individuals involved in the healthcare industry, from medical practitioners to students.

The scope and constraints of the book are clearly stated, giving readers a clear idea of the bounds and breadth of content. In-depth discussion of pulmonary embolism's definition, synopsis, and the structure and operation of the lungs are provided in Chapter 1. The etiology, pathophysiology, clinical presentation, diagnostic techniques, therapeutic choices, preventive measures, consequences, and long-term repercussions of pulmonary embolism are all thoroughly explained in the following chapters.

The focus on patient education and assistance in Chapter 8 is especially noteworthy. Understanding how important it is to arm patients with information, the book discusses lifestyle modifications, treatment adherence, and the availability of services and support groups. This all-encompassing strategy guarantees that patients and medical professionals can both actively engage in managing and preventing pulmonary embolism, improving the general state of healthcare.

As a fundamental work in the medical literature, "Pulmonary Embolism" provides a comprehensive analysis of the ailment and is a priceless tool for anybody researching, diagnosing, or treating pulmonary embolism.

Introduction

A dangerous medical disorder known as pulmonary embolism (PE) is characterized by an abrupt obstruction of one or more pulmonary arteries in the lungs. Deep vein thrombosis (DVT), a disorder where blood clots migrate from deep veins in the legs to the lungs, is usually the cause of this obstruction. PE is a potentially fatal illness, so it's important for researchers, medical experts, and even the general public to comprehend all of its nuances. This thorough analysis explores the book's goal, highlighting the significance of understanding pulmonary embolism, determining the intended audience, and admitting the study's limits.

Objective Of The Book

This book's main goal is to give readers a thorough understanding of pulmonary embolism, including information on its pathophysiology, methods of diagnosis, and available treatments.

The book intends to be a useful tool for healthcare professionals, such as doctors, nurses, and allied health workers, who want to improve their proficiency in treating patients with pulmonary embolism by combining the most recent research and practical information. It also offers a thorough examination of the complexity of the illness, making it a useful teaching tool for medical students and residents. In addition, the book aims to close the knowledge gap between scientific studies and real-world applications, promoting a comprehensive awareness of pulmonary embolism among medical professionals.

Comprehending Pulmonary Embolism Is Crucial

Because pulmonary embolism can be fatal and has a major influence on public health, it is crucial to understand this condition. PE continues to be the primary cause of morbidity and death globally and is responsible for a significant portion of hospital admissions.

Through a thorough exploration of the etiology, risk factors, and clinical symptoms, medical professionals can enhance their ability to identify and treat this disorder. Furthermore, a deeper comprehension of PE makes it easier to create focused preventative plans and cutting-edge therapy therapies, both of which eventually improve patient outcomes.

Public awareness of PE's symptoms and indicators is also increased by education, which makes early detection and prompt intervention possible.

The Intended Audience

This book is designed to fulfill the informational requirements of a wide range of medical professionals. The information is relevant to the specializations of cardiologists, pulmonologists, emergency medicine doctors, radiologists, and vascular surgeons, among other healthcare experts. Comprehensive coverage will be beneficial to medical students and residents who wish to expand their understanding of cardiovascular and pulmonary disorders. Additionally, practical insights to improve clinical skills will be provided for nurses and other allied health professionals involved in the care of patients with pulmonary embolism.

The book is a useful resource for academics and researchers working on cardiovascular issues because it provides a summary of the available data and suggests possible directions for further investigation.

Range And Restrictions

This book covers a wide range of subjects about pulmonary embolism, such as its epidemiology, pathophysiology, clinical manifestation, diagnostic techniques, and treatment approaches.

An extensive examination of risk factors, prophylaxis, and emerging research adds to the content's comprehensiveness. But it's important to recognize the limitations that come with any medical literature.

There may occasionally be gaps in the coverage of the most recent advancements due to the quickly changing field of medical research. Additionally, practitioners should always take patient-specific considerations into account while making therapeutic decisions.

The book does not substitute personalized medical advice.

Notwithstanding these drawbacks, the book offers a strong framework for comprehending pulmonary embolism and encourages readers to go further into the subject through additional study and hands-on training.

CHAPTER ONE
FUNDAMENTALS OF PULMONARY EMBOLISM

A dangerous medical disorder known as pulmonary embolism (PE) is characterized by an abrupt obstruction of one or more pulmonary arteries in the lungs. Usually, embolism—a condition in which blood clots from deep veins in the legs or other regions of the body migrate to the lungs—causes this obstruction. PE is a potentially fatal illness that needs to be diagnosed and treated right away to avoid serious side effects including respiratory failure or even death.

Overview Of Empathy

Understanding embolism in general is crucial to understanding pulmonary embolism.

Any substance that enters the bloodstream and becomes lodged in a blood artery, blocking blood flow, is called an embolus. When a pulmonary embolism occurs, a blood clot typically forms in the deep veins of the legs. The clot then breaks off and travels down the veins to the lungs. There could be catastrophic repercussions if there is an abrupt blockage in the pulmonary arteries that prevents blood from reaching the lungs.

Pulmonary Embolism Types

Based on the size and place of origin of the embolus, pulmonary emboli can be categorized into different categories. Thromboembolism is the most common variety, in which a thrombus, or blood clot, forms in a deep vein, usually in the leg, and proceeds to the lungs. Although less frequent, fat, air, and amniotic fluid emboli can also result in pulmonary embolism. Understanding the variations between each kind is essential for a precise diagnosis and suitable therapy. Each type has unique traits.

The Lungs' Anatomy And Function

It is essential to comprehend the structure and operation of the lungs in order to fully appreciate the effects of pulmonary embolism. The lungs are essential organs that remove carbon dioxide from the blood and oxygenate it. From the heart, deoxygenated blood is transported via the pulmonary arteries to the lungs, where oxygen is exchanged for carbon dioxide. Any blockage in these arteries, like a pulmonary embolism, interferes with this vital exchange, resulting in a reduced flow of oxygen and possibly serious implications for the body as a whole.

Circulation Of The Pulmonary

The circulatory system that moves blood from the heart to the lungs is called pulmonary circulation. Blood flows easily via the pulmonary arteries in a healthy circulatory system, facilitating effective oxygenation.

This circulation is upset by pulmonary embolism, which results in an abrupt obstruction that impairs the lungs' capacity to oxygenate blood. To understand how and why pulmonary embolism can have such severe impacts on respiratory and cardiovascular function, one must have a thorough understanding of the complexities of pulmonary circulation.

The Function Of Coagulation

Coagulation, or the process of blood clotting, is essential for preserving hemostasis and limiting excessive bleeding. Nevertheless, dysregulation of this process can result in aberrant blood clot formation, which is a common cause of pulmonary embolism. Blood clots can form due to various factors, including heredity, underlying medical disorders, or extended immobility. Investigating the complex processes involved in blood clotting is essential for determining risk factors and putting preventative measures in place to avoid pulmonary embolism.

Risk Elements For Heart Attack

For the purposes of early detection and prevention, a thorough understanding of the risk factors linked to pulmonary embolism is essential.

Deep vein thrombosis (DVT), a disorder where blood clots form in the deep veins, mainly in the legs, is one of the common risk factors.

Additional risk factors include trauma, surgery, extended immobility, pregnancy, and specific medical problems such clotting disorders and cancer.

By identifying these risk factors, medical personnel can identify patients who are more likely to experience a pulmonary embolism and take preventive action.

DVT, Or Deep Vein Thrombosis

One of the main risk factors for many pulmonary embolism occurrences is deep vein thrombosis (DVT). Blood clots in the deep veins, generally in the legs, cause DVT. A pulmonary embolism can result from these clots dislodging and moving through the bloodstream and into the lungs. It is crucial to comprehend the pathophysiology of deep vein thrombosis (DVT) in order to identify the initial symptoms and indicators of the condition and to put treatments in place that stop DVT from developing into a potentially fatal pulmonary embolism.

Additional Contributing Elements

In addition to DVT, there are a plethora of additional factors that raise the risk of pulmonary embolism. People who have had surgery, especially orthopedic and cancer surgeries, are more likely to develop blood clots. Moreover, trauma from severe injuries or fractures may have a role in the formation of emboli. Furthermore, pulmonary embolism risk may be elevated by medical illnesses such as heart failure, inflammatory disorders, and atrial fibrillation. Developing customized preventative efforts and identifying high-risk populations are made easier with a thorough investigation of these relevant factors.

In order to fully comprehend pulmonary embolism, one must examine its definition, the definition of embolism as a whole, its different forms, the structure and operation of the lungs, pulmonary circulation, blood clotting, risk factors, the importance of deep vein thrombosis, and other relevant factors. Healthcare providers must use this comprehensive strategy for diagnosing, treating, and preventing pulmonary embolism in order to improve patient outcomes and lower the high morbidity and fatality rates connected to this serious illness.

CHAPTER TWO
ORIGINS AND PATHOPHYSIOLOGY

A dangerous medical illness known as pulmonary embolism (PE) is defined by pulmonary artery blockage, typically brought on by blood clots. Effective diagnosis, prevention, and treatment of PE depend on an understanding of its pathophysiology and etiology.

The Cause And Development Of Blood Clots

Thrombi, or blood clots that form inside the circulatory system, are frequently the cause of pulmonary embolism. Deep vein thrombosis (DVT) is the term for the condition where thrombi usually begin in the deep veins of the lower limbs.

People are predisposed to the formation of these clots due to the complex interaction of Virchow's triad, which includes blood stasis, hypercoagulability, and vascular endothelial damage. Endothelial damage, frequently brought on by trauma or surgery, prepares the body for the production of clots. Furthermore, a hypercoagulable state can be exacerbated by diseases including cancer, genetic predispositions, and hormonal variables, which increases the likelihood of thrombus formation.

Common Reasons For Heart Attacks

1 Deep vein thrombosis:

Thrombosis in the body's deep veins, especially in the lower limbs, is one of the main causes of pulmonary embolism. Long-term immobilization, surgery, trauma, and other conditions can disturb normal blood flow and cause stasis, which raises the risk of thrombus formation. A potentially fatal pulmonary embolism can occur if a piece of this thrombus breaks off and travels through the bloodstream to lodge in the pulmonary arteries.

2 Assimilation from Different Websites:

Other materials than thrombi can also embolize and cause pulmonary embolism. Other than blood clots, other materials can restrict blood flow in the pulmonary circulation through emboli such as fat, air, or amniotic fluid. Fat globules are released into the bloodstream during traumatic injuries or some orthopedic surgeries, and this might cause embolism by traveling to the pulmonary arteries.

<u>The Pathophysiological Mechanisms:</u>

<u>One Migration of Blood Clots:</u>

One important step in the pathogenesis of pulmonary embolism is the migration of blood clots from their place of origin into the pulmonary vasculature. An embolus forms when a thrombus separates from the deep veins and moves through the venous system to the right side of the heart. The embolus may be launched into the pulmonary artery from the right atrium, obstructing it.

The severity of the pulmonary embolism is determined by the embolus's size and the level of occlusion it causes.

Effect No. 2 on the Pulmonary Vasculature

A pulmonary embolism has aftereffects that go beyond the original mechanical restriction. Acute right heart strain is caused by an increase in pulmonary vascular resistance following an abrupt blockage of the pulmonary arteries.

Acute cor pulmonale is the term for this phenomenon, which can cause right ventricular failure and dysfunction. A series of inflammatory reactions and vasoconstriction are set off by the blocked blood flow, worsening the condition of the lungs' perfusion.

Hypoxemia is a result of mismatches between ventilation and perfusion in afflicted lung areas, which can lead to respiratory failure.

The mechanism and causes of pulmonary embolism must be thoroughly understood by doctors, researchers, and healthcare professionals.

It permits the creation of focused diagnostic plans, prophylactic actions, and treatment plans to lessen the morbidity and death resulting from this dangerous vascular condition.

CHAPTER THREE
CLINICAL PRESENTATION

The potentially fatal illness known as pulmonary embolism (PE) is defined by the abrupt obstruction of one or more pulmonary arteries by emboli, which are primarily blood clots that originate from the legs' deep veins. Pulmonary embolism can show in a variety of ways clinically, therefore prompt and precise diagnosis is essential for the best course of treatment. PE symptoms can be divided into three categories: cardiovascular, respiratory, and other related symptoms.

<u>Symptoms and Indications:</u>

1 Symptoms of the Respiration:

Patients who have experienced a pulmonary embolism frequently have respiratory symptoms, which are indicative of reduced blood supply to the lungs. One of the main symptoms is dyspnea, or shortness of breath, which can be minor or severe depending on the size and location of the embolus. Pleuritic chest discomfort that is limited to the damaged lung area and worsens with breathing is a possible symptom for patients. The body may try to make up for the decreased oxygenation by causing tachypnea and hyperventilation. In certain situations, another respiratory indication that may be seen is hemoptysis, or coughing up blood-streaked sputum.

2. symptoms of heart disease:

Because of the effect on heart function, people with pulmonary embolism frequently experience cardiovascular symptoms. A common result is tachycardia, which is the body's reaction to the decreased oxygen flow. Different from pleuritic discomfort, chest pain can happen and is commonly described as a stabbing or sharp feeling. In extreme situations, people may experience hepatomegaly, peripheral edema, and increased jugular vein pressure—all indicators of right heart strain. In the event of a major pulmonary embolism, hypotension may develop, which can cause shock and hemodynamic instability.

Three Additional Related Symptoms

Patients who have a pulmonary embolism may also experience a wide range of other related symptoms in addition to respiratory and cardiovascular issues. Because of the general load on the circulatory system and the decreased oxygen delivery to tissues, fatigue and weakness are typical. There may also be reports of lightheadedness and sweating. Even though it is less common, syncope can happen, particularly when there is a large pulmonary embolism and there is an abrupt and noticeable decrease in cardiac output.

Diagnostic Differentiation:

.1 Differentiating Between Heart Attack and Other Conditions:

Because pulmonary embolism shares clinical features with a number of other illnesses, the differential diagnosis must be carefully considered. The diagnostic process can be difficult because conditions like myocardial infarction, pneumonia, and exacerbations of chronic obstructive pulmonary disease (COPD) may have similar symptoms.

Although dyspnea and pleuritic chest pain are common respiratory symptoms of pneumonia, a thorough clinical and radiological evaluation can help distinguish it from pulmonary embolism. Different therapeutic techniques are needed for chest pain and dyspnea, two symptoms that can be indicative of myocardial infarction. It is critical to distinguish between the two. Dyspnea and coughing are common symptoms of COPD exacerbations, and a complete medical history and physical examination are necessary for a precise diagnosis.

The diagnosis of pulmonary embolism can be confirmed or ruled out with the use of imaging studies such as echocardiography, ventilation-perfusion (V/Q) scanning, and computed tomography pulmonary angiography (CTPA). Correct diagnosis and adequate care (anticoagulation therapy or more invasive measures in severe cases) depend on the integration of clinical judgment, risk stratification techniques, and imaging data.

there is variation in the clinical manifestation of pulmonary embolism, encompassing respiratory, cardiovascular, and additional related symptoms. For prompt and efficient treatment, it is critical to identify the symptoms and indicators of pulmonary embolism and conduct a thorough differential diagnosis to distinguish it from other illnesses. In the setting of this potentially fatal illness, correct diagnosis and optimal patient outcomes depend on the integration of modern imaging techniques and clinical evaluation.

CHAPTER FOUR
DIAGNOSTIC METHODS

Different diagnostic techniques are used in the quest for an accurate diagnosis of adult acute myeloid leukemia (AML). Each strategy provides vital information that helps clinicians in their assessment and subsequent management of the disease.

Imaging Methodologies

Imaging is essential to the diagnosis of AML because it helps to visualize possible side effects and provides information about how the illness is progressing. One such method is pulmonary angiography, which involves injecting contrast material into the pulmonary arteries in order to find any irregularities in the flow of blood. This process is very helpful in identifying thrombotic events or leukemic infiltrates in the pulmonary vasculature.

An further imaging method that improves the visibility of the pulmonary arteries and provides detailed cross-sectional pictures is

CT pulmonary angiography. This method offers a more thorough evaluation of the vascular anomalies linked to AML, assisting in the detection of thromboembolic episodes and directing therapeutic choices.

Ventilation-Perfusion Scans are useful for assessing lung health and identifying anomalies in the lungs' blood perfusion and ventilation.

These scans can aid in the identification of pulmonary problems related to AML, such as leukemic infiltrates or emboli, which can lead to a more comprehensive understanding of the disease's effect on respiratory function.

Laboratory Examinations

Laboratory testing are essential for verifying the AML diagnosis and determining how much the disease has affected different physiological markers. Measuring the amount of fibrin breakdown products in the blood, the D-dimer test is useful in detecting hypercoagulable conditions and thrombotic events linked to AML. Increased D-dimer levels could lead to more research into possible side effects and influence treatment choices.

Vital signs concerning the patient's respiratory and metabolic conditions are provided by the blood gas analysis. This test aids in determining how the illness affects gas exchange and acid-base balance in the context of AML. Blood gas parameter abnormalities can impact the overall care plan by pointing to respiratory distress or other problems.

the diagnostic methods for adult acute myeloid leukemia employ a multimodal approach that integrates laboratory testing and imaging modalities to offer a thorough grasp of the illness's symptoms. Insights into vascular and respiratory difficulties can be gained by pulmonary angiography, CT pulmonary angiography, and ventilation-perfusion scans.

Important data regarding coagulation status and physiological parameters can be obtained from the D-dimer test and blood gas analysis.

The amalgamation of various diagnostic methods augments the accuracy of AML diagnosis and expedites a focused therapeutic intervention strategy.

CHAPTER FIVE
AVAILABLE TREATMENTS

A complicated class of diseases known as amyloidosis is defined by the aberrant build-up of misfolded proteins, or amyloids, in different human tissues and organs. Because of the condition's heterogeneity and potential involvement of important systems such the liver, heart, kidneys, and nervous system, it presents a considerable challenge. The management of amyloidosis and the reduction of its accompanying symptoms have changed along with our understanding of the illness. This section explores the range of therapeutic options available, such as pain management, cardiac and renal supportive care, targeted medicines, chemotherapy, and stem cell transplantation. It also discusses symptomatic management.

One of the most important aspects of treating amyloidosis is chemotherapy, especially when systemic involvement is visible.

Chemotherapeutic drugs are used to specifically target and eradicate the aberrant plasma cells that produce amyloid fibrils. Notably, medications like dexamethasone and melphalan have shown promise in treating specific types of amyloidosis, including light-chain (AL) amyloidosis. Chemotherapy selection is contingent upon the particular subtype and level of organ involvement. Chemotherapy has the ability to control the disease and relieve symptoms, but there are risks that must be carefully considered, and patients must be closely monitored.

For suitable patients with amyloidosis, stem cell transplantation (SCT) stands out as a more aggressive therapy approach. In this surgery, healthy stem cells—typically obtained from the patient or a suitable donor—replace the damaged bone marrow.

The use of the patient's own stem cells in autologous stem cell transplantation has showed promise in the treatment of AL amyloidosis. Allogeneic stem cell transplantation, which uses donor stem cells, is only used in specific circumstances because of the increased risks and problems involved. With proper patient selection, stem cell transplantation (SCT) offers a potentially curative strategy by stopping the generation of amyloidogenic proteins and restoring normal hematopoiesis.

Treatment options for amyloidosis have completely changed with the advent of targeted medicines, which provide more specialized and less hazardous options. Monoclonal antibodies that target plasma cells and prevent the development of amyloid fibrils, like daratumumab and ixazomib, have shown promise in treating AL amyloidosis.

Protease inhibitors, such as bortezomib, have also demonstrated potential in lowering amyloid buildup.

In addition to offering brand-new therapeutic alternatives, these targeted medicines advance personalized medicine by enabling more specialized strategies based on the underlying molecular and genetic traits of the amyloidosis subtype.

In addition to treatments aimed at altering the course of the disease, effective symptom management is essential for improving the quality of life for those who have amyloidosis.

Given that amyloidosis frequently involves the heart, cardiac supportive care is crucial. Medication for heart failure, such as beta-blockers and diuretics, can be used as part of management efforts to enhance cardiac function and reduce symptoms. Heart transplantation may be considered in extreme instances.

The problems caused by amyloid buildup in the kidneys, which frequently results in proteinuria and renal failure, are addressed by renal supportive treatment.

Treatment for renal problems often involves blood pressure regulation, ACE inhibitors, and angiotensin II receptor blockers (ARBs).

An essential part of the total care plan for people with amyloidosis is pain control. Neuropathic pain, which arises from amyloid buildup in peripheral nerves, necessitates a multidisciplinary approach to treat pain's emotional and sensory components. It is possible to use neuropathic painkillers like gabapentin and pregabalin in addition to physical treatment and psychological support.

An integrated approach to symptom control also includes measures for managing organ-specific symptoms connected to amyloid, such as autonomic dysfunction or gastrointestinal problems.

there are many different approaches to treating amyloidosis, which reflects the variety of symptoms and underlying pathophysiology of this intricate illness. Traditional chemotherapy and novel targeted medicines are available as treatment options; stem cell transplantation may be able to cure some people. Managing symptoms, especially those related to heart and kidney problems, is essential to enhancing the lives of those with amyloidosis. Future improvements in effectiveness and individualization are anticipated as research yields new insights into the mechanisms underlying the disease and therapy options continue to evolve.

CHAPTER SIX
STRATEGIES FOR PREVENTION

A dangerous medical illness known as pulmonary embolism (PE) is characterized by the abrupt obstruction of one or more pulmonary arteries in the lungs. Blood clots that originate in the legs or other parts of the body are typically the source of PE. One of the most important aspects of patient care is preventing pulmonary embolism (PE).

To reduce the risk of deep vein thrombosis (DVT), which frequently precedes PE, a number of techniques are used. The prevention techniques for PE will be covered in detail in this section, with particular attention paid to pharmaceutical methods, mechanical prophylaxis, dietary considerations, and lifestyle changes that include physical activity and exercise.

One essential component of preventing pulmonary embolism is the prevention of deep vein thrombosis.

Pharmacological methods entail the administration of anticoagulant drugs to prevent the formation of blood clots. These drugs, which include warfarin and heparin, lower the risk of thrombus formation in the deep veins by blocking particular clotting factors. To choose the best anticoagulant regimen, doctors carefully review patient profiles, taking into account things like age, medical history, and existing drugs. Despite the great efficacy of these drugs, careful observation is necessary to avoid side effects including severe bleeding.

In the fight against DVT, mechanical prophylaxis is just as important as pharmaceutical methods. In order to improve blood circulation and avoid stagnation in the deep veins, compression stockings or intermittent pneumatic compression devices are used. By applying pressure to the legs, compression stockings help to avoid blood clots and pooling of blood.

Conversely, intermittent pneumatic compression devices periodically inflate and deflate to replicate the calf muscles' normal pumping function.

These techniques are especially helpful for people who are at a higher risk of developing DVT, such as those who are having surgery or will be immobile for extended periods of time.

Making changes to one's lifestyle is another important aspect of PE prevention.

Physical activity and regular exercise are essential for lowering the risk of DVT. Engaging in physical activity stimulates blood flow and averts stasis by strengthening the muscles, especially the lower limbs. Including exercises like swimming, cycling, or walking in one's regimen can make a big difference in one's vascular health.

A healthy weight and a non-sedentary lifestyle are also crucial aspects in changing one's way of living. Since obesity increases the risk of DVT, controlling weight is an essential preventive approach.

The prevention of pulmonary embolism is also influenced by dietary factors. Dietary factors can have an impact on vascular health and blood clotting. Drinking enough water keeps the blood from getting too thick, which lowers the risk of clot formation. A diet high in fruits, vegetables, and whole grains also contributes to general cardiovascular health by providing vital nutrients and antioxidants. Conversely, consuming too many meals high in cholesterol and saturated fats can worsen atherosclerosis and raise the risk of blood clots. A balanced, heart-healthy diet is typically emphasized by medical practitioners in addition to other preventive measures.

To sum up, preventing pulmonary embolism requires a multimodal strategy that includes lifestyle, mechanical, and pharmaceutical measures. Deep vein thrombosis must be prevented as much as possible. Pharmacological prophylaxis uses anticoagulant drugs, while mechanical prophylaxis uses compression stockings or intermittent pneumatic compression devices. A heart-healthy diet, consistent exercise, and weight control are all essential elements in the prevention of PE. Healthcare professionals emphasize the significance of a thorough and individualized approach to reduce the risk of deep vein thrombosis, which is a precursor to pulmonary embolism, and customize preventative strategies based on specific patient profiles.

CHAPTER SEVEN
INTRICACIES AND PROLONGED CONSEQUENCES

A dangerous and sometimes fatal medical illness known as pulmonary embolism (PE) is characterized by blockage of the pulmonary arteries, which is typically brought on by blood clots that make their way from deep veins in the legs or other regions of the body to the lungs. Although PE's immediate effects are widely known and frequently treated right away, the condition's long-term ramifications and complications also need careful thought.

Chronic Thromboembolic Pulmonary Hypertension (CTEPH): The development of chronic thromboembolic pulmonary hypertension (CTEPH) is one of the major long-term consequences of pulmonary embolism. A rare but severe kind of pulmonary hypertension known as CTEPH develops when blood clots do not fully disintegrate, causing the pulmonary arteries to remain persistently blocked. This may eventually lead to right heart strain, elevated pulmonary vascular resistance, and heart failure.

A difficult component of managing PE is CTEPH, which calls for specific diagnostic techniques like pulmonary angiography and, in extreme circumstances, surgical procedures like pulmonary endarterectomy.

The term "Post-Pulmonary Embolism Syndrome" (PES) refers to a group of problems and aftereffects that may last for a considerable amount of time following an acute episode of PE. Persistent respiratory symptoms, such as dyspnea, coughing, and decreased exercise tolerance, are one facet of PES. These symptoms, which are frequently ascribed to the aftereffects of the initial embolic event, can be a sign of continuing lung parenchymal and vascular damage. It takes thorough monitoring and follow-up to find and treat these enduring respiratory problems.

Persistent Respiratory Symptoms: A typical indicator of PES, persistent respiratory symptoms can have a serious negative effect on a person's quality of life after suffering a pulmonary embolism. Breathlessness, or dyspnea, is a characteristic symptom that can last for a long time because of problems with lung mechanics or pulmonary function. Chest pain is frequently associated with coughing, which can linger and add to the total burden of respiratory distress. Targeted therapy approaches, such as pulmonary rehabilitation, bronchodilators, or anticoagulant regimens customized to address persistent vascular abnormalities, may be necessary to manage these symptoms, which can be incapacitating.

Problems with Quality of Life: Pulmonary embolism can result in a wide range of problems with quality of life in addition to physiological difficulties. In addition to the persistent physical symptoms, the psychological effects of surviving a life-threatening event can result in worry, despair, and a general decline in wellbeing. Patients could find it difficult to resume their prior level of physical activity and might find it difficult to go about their everyday lives. Psychological support, patient education, and comprehensive rehabilitation programs are essential components in treating the complex quality of life problems related to pulmonary embolism.

pulmonary embolism is a disorder that can have long-term effects in addition to being an immediate medical issue. Comprehensive and multidisciplinary care techniques are necessary for conditions including post-pulmonary embolism syndrome and chronic thromboembolic pulmonary hypertension, which include persistent respiratory symptoms and problems with quality of life.

A comprehensive approach to treating patients who have had a pulmonary embolism must acknowledge and manage these consequences, placing equal emphasis on survival and the return of the patient's body to its best.

CHAPTER EIGHT
EDUCATION AND SUPPORT FOR PATIENTS

The sudden obstruction of one or more pulmonary arteries in the lungs is known as pulmonary embolism (PE), a dangerous medical illness that is usually brought on by blood clots that migrate from the legs or other parts of the body to the lungs. Comprehensive patient education and support, in addition to medical measures, are essential for the effective management of pulmonary embolism. In order to maximize treatment results, avoid recurrence, and enhance the general quality of life for those afflicted with this potentially fatal illness, a comprehensive approach is needed.

Patient Education: An essential part of patient empowerment and self-management, patient education is a cornerstone in the therapy of pulmonary embolism. In order to promote informed decision-making and improve treatment compliance, it is imperative that patients receive comprehensive education regarding the nature of pulmonary embolism, its risk factors, and potential sequelae. Patients should be made aware of the warning signs and symptoms of PE, which include fast heartbeat, chest discomfort, and shortness of breath, so they can seek immediate medical assistance if needed. Preventing repeated thromboembolic episodes also requires educating patients about the significance of taking anticoagulant drugs as prescribed and scheduling follow-up sessions.

Comprehensive education should cover long-term consequences as well as the danger of persistent problems such chronic thromboembolic pulmonary hypertension (CTEPH), in addition to the immediate pulmonary embolism crisis. To actively engage in their care, patients must understand the logic behind treatment plans, possible drug side effects, and lifestyle changes. Effective communication between healthcare providers and patients, along with the provision of written materials, can enhance the learning process and guarantee that patients have the necessary information to make well-informed decisions regarding their health.

Lifestyle Modifications and Treatment Adherence: Changing one's lifestyle is essential for managing and preventing pulmonary emboli. Anticoagulant drugs, such as warfarin or direct oral anticoagulants (DOACs), are frequently administered to patients with PE in order to stop additional clot formation. It is imperative to comprehend the significance of medication adherence, since noncompliance with therapy can result in treatment failure and a heightened risk of subsequent thromboembolic events. Patients should be informed by their healthcare professionals about how to take drugs correctly, possible drug interactions, and the value of routine monitoring to keep therapeutic anticoagulation levels at bay.

Lifestyle modifications are essential for lowering the risk of recurrent pulmonary embolism and improving general cardiovascular health, in addition to medication adherence. Patients should receive counseling on leading a healthy lifestyle that includes giving up smoking, eating a balanced diet, and getting frequent exercise. Given that obesity is a known risk factor for venous thromboembolism, weight management is very crucial. Additionally, patients need to be informed about the ways to reduce their risk of clot formation as well as the possible effects of specific activities, like extended immobility during lengthy flights.

Support Groups and Resources: Because pulmonary embolisms can have a profound emotional and psychological impact on patients, support groups and resources are important sources of support and coping skills. A pulmonary embolism can be a distressing event that frequently results in worry about recurrence, sadness, and anxiety. Online or in-person support groups provide a forum for patients to talk about their struggles, ask for guidance, and get emotional support from like-minded people.

Healthcare professionals should tell patients about available services and actively encourage them to join support groups. These support groups provide useful practical information on living with pulmonary embolism in addition to providing emotional support. Patient education stresses the value of mental and emotional health while addressing the individual's overall well-being, going beyond the clinical components of the illness.

Healthcare providers should direct patients to reliable educational resources, both online and offline, in addition to support groups. Websites, brochures, and instructional materials from medical groups that focus on cardiovascular health may fall under this category. Giving patients access to trustworthy information improves their capacity to take an active role in their care, make wise decisions, and speak up for their own interests.

a thorough strategy for treating pulmonary embolism must include patient education and support.

Healthcare practitioners may help patients with this potentially fatal condition live healthier lives and achieve better results by stressing the value of patient education, encouraging lifestyle modifications, and putting them in touch with resources and support groups. This all-encompassing strategy takes into account the patients' long-term resilience and well-being in the face of pulmonary embolism and its aftermath in addition to attending to their urgent medical demands.

CONCLUSION

pulmonary embolism is a complicated, potentially fatal illness with a wide range of clinical manifestations and consequences. Healthcare practitioners caring for patients with this condition must possess a comprehensive awareness of its pathogenesis, risk factors, clinical symptoms, diagnostic techniques, treatment strategies, and long-term results. The management of pulmonary embolism is always changing due to advancements in diagnostic techniques and available treatments, which highlights the significance of continuing research and patient education in enhancing outcomes.

A comprehensive and patient-centered approach is still essential to provide the best care and averting the catastrophic effects of pulmonary embolism as we traverse the complexity of this illness.